Natural Weight Loss Hypnosis

Lose Weight with Hypnosis, Meditation and Affirmations

Written By

Guided Meditation Therapy

Table of Contents

Introduction

Do you struggle to lose weight? Have you always visualized yourself as thin, attractive, and free from any health conditions brought on by excess weight? Do you desire to get certain things in your life, only to feel held back by the body that you have?

Sometimes, we struggle to lose weight because we don't have the right mindset to do so. We expect doing physical things like eating healthy and exercising to be all that it takes. A huge part of weight loss is psychological. In fact, this might be the most important part of all. If you don't have a healthy mindset and one that is focused on getting better, then you might struggle to actually lose the weight. Not only this, but you might find that you struggle because you can't keep the weight off, even after you lose it initially.

Throughout this book, we have provided you with four different mindset exercises in order to help you lose weight. These are hypnosis, meditations, and affirmations that will make it easier for you to rewire your brain so that you're focused on achieving your goals and getting the things that you want from this life.

Make sure that you do not do any of these meditations while you're driving or operating a motor vehicle. The best place possible for these meditations is in your home, in a place where you are completely relaxed and at ease. You do not want to put yourself in a risky situation by doing this meditation somewhere that you can't fall asleep. After you know how you react to these meditations, you might be able to do them in public, such as riding a train or an airplane for long periods of travel. However, ensure that you understand how you might react, especially to hypnosis. Make sure that, as you're reading or listening to these meditations, you are focused on your breath, and keep an open mind. Letting your thoughts flow free can be the key to ensuring that you get the healthy body that you deserve.

Chapter 1: Meditation for Weight Loss

One of the hardest parts about losing weight is having to wait so long to see the results. While there isn't a way to lose 20 pounds overnight, you can reshape your mentality so that you can grow your patience for the process. When you fully recognize time and how that plays into weight loss, you won't be looking at the scale every hour, begging for results. Instead, you will be happy with your journey and able to recognize the incredible way that your body is changing. This is a visualization exercise that is going to help you get in the right mindset to lose weight fast.

Fast Weight Loss Meditation

This meditation is going to be a visualization. You are going to want to make sure that you are in a comfortable place where you can drift off and go to sleep if you want to. We are going to take you through the scene that will await you at the end of your natural weight loss journey. We often have many ideas of what we want to get from our weight loss process, but we don't always visualize what the actual setting could be. In this meditation, we are going to help you understand the realistic scenario that you could find yourself in after you've managed to lose the weight. Close your eyes and keep your body as relaxed as possible. Start to focus on your breathing. Breathe in through your nose and out through your mouth. Concentrate the air as it travels through your body so that you will be able to shut out any negative or toxic thoughts more easily than you have in this moment.

Focus on your breathing and breathe in for five and out for five. We are going to count down through 10 a few times in order to get you in the right mindset.

Breathe in now for one, two, three, four, and five, and out for five, four, three, two, and one.

Now we are going to count down from 10. Make sure that you are still focused on breathing in this pattern.

Ten, nine, eight, seven, six, five, four, three, two, and one.

You see nothing around you. Everything is black, and you are completely relaxed.

Each time a new thought comes into your brain, simply push it out and focus instead on your breathing. Again, breathe in for one, two, three, four, and five, and out for five, four, three, two, and one.

You are now completely relaxed. There is nothing in front of you. Your eyes are closed and you only see black. Everything is dark and peaceful. You don't have to worry about anything in this moment.

Nothing is around you.

You are completely quiet and totally serene. Your body is feeling free and relaxed. You look ahead of you and you start to see a little white dot. This white continues to grow and grow and grow until it has engulfed you.

You see a perfectly clear blue sky with the sun shining down. The white comes from the bright gravel driveway that's in front of you. You start to walk towards a gigantic mansion. You take a few steps up and notice the marble front doors in front of you. You are looking out, and you see nothing but a green grassy pasture and skyline dotted with trees. You are completely centered and peaceful in this moment. You reach your hand out and grasp the brass knob right in front of you. You squeeze it gently and turn it, slowly pushing the door open. You feel the cool air come out as you take a big deep breath in and take a step. In front of you is an amazing wooden carved staircase with marble furnishings. The floor is an ornate tile with intricate designs. You look up and see that there is a gorgeous sunroof letting a beam of light hit you like an angel.

You close the door behind you and take your settings in once more. This mansion is yours. You recognize now that this is your very own home. You take a step forward, and you notice there's a mirror against the wall. You walk towards the mirror and see yourself standing there, only this isn't the self that you know now as you are in this present moment. This is somebody who has naturally lost the weight.

Your body is pure and healthy. You don't have any marks from surgeries or the sign of starvation in your eyes. You are happy because you have completed this task naturally. You worked alongside your body in order to get the results that you not only want but also deserve. You look around you and see that you have managed to create this life. You have your dream body with your dream hair and a happy shining face, and you are surrounded by everything you could ever want. You notice there's a long hallway, and you hear some chatter at the end. Before following you stop first into a bedroom against a long hallway. On the bed, you see the most gorgeous outfit you could ever imagine. It has all the makings of something that not only helps you to look good but makes you feel good. You slip into this outfit now and take a look in the mirror. Once again, your incredibly defined body shows through this silhouette. You exude confidence. It really doesn't even matter what you're wearing, but this outfit, in particular, makes you feel like a luxury.

You start to admire your body from the bottom up. You notice your incredible feet and how they have been able to carry you throughout this whole process. You have shoes that comfortably fit, and your body is no longer sore. You can easily move your ankles and your feet around as needed. They carry you to places that you never thought you would find yourself. They have been able to hold your entire body. Without these powerful feet, you would not have been able to go through this whole process. You move on up now to your calves. You see these intense calves combined with your shins and understand the way that they have helped to also push you forward. You were able to run and walk on these calves to burn so many calories. You naturally used this small part of your body to have so much powerful force.

You were able to lift weights; and you were able to do squats, jumping jacks, and other fun exercises. They help you dance. Each time you move your calf, you notice that this is something so powerful and strong. That really helped you through this journey. Moving up, you see your knees and your thighs. This part helped you bend, and you were able to stretch and feel your muscles relax as you worked them out.

You're able to recognize all of the powerful and incredible ways that your legs have carried you throughout this life. They have helped you to run, exercise, and jog, along with other methods of physical exercise, so that you are able to get the body that you desire. These incredible legs look so great in the mirror as you look in front of you. You are not afraid to show them off anymore. They are a part of who you are. You see your stomach now, and it shows just how incredibly strong your willpower is. You've been able to say no to food that you know not only adds extra weight to your body but just generally makes you feel bad. You don't have that big gut anymore that is filled with foods that are unhealthy. Having a belly is not bad at all. Most animals even need this belly. However, your gut isn't one that weighs you down. You don't feel so full and greasy in your stomach. You feel good. You know that you've been working with your gut in a healthy and happy way to provide it with everything that it needs. You haven't been feeding it food that makes it feel bad. You only give it good nutritious food that is easy for it to process. It breaks down your food and takes every mineral, vitamin, and nutrient from this substance in order to make you feel better. Your stomach knows exactly what to do with food and where to send the various parts that it breaks down as well.

You look up and see your incredible chest.

This has been where your heart beats and your lungs work hard during your workouts. These organs work so efficiently because your stomach was able to process everything that you fed it for a long period of time. Your chest is where the center of your body lies. You are able to look at this incredible tool and see the way that you've been able to transform your body. You feel yourself breathe in again as you notice how it rises and falls with each breath that you take.

Breathe in for one, two, three, four, and five, and out for five, four, three, two, and one.

You keep breathing, and your heart keeps pumping. Even when you're sleeping or not even thinking about it, your heart and lungs will continue to work. This has been an incredibly powerful part of your journey. You look in the mirror and notice your arms. These powerful and strong arms have also helped to carry you through this process.

They did the push-ups, the pull-ups, and everything else in between. They helped prepare your delicious food. Your hands were able to make things that helped you to feel better in this life. Your arms are what carried you throughout your journey.

You were able to hold yourself. You could massage your muscles, and you soothe yourself using your hands. These are so powerful and a part of this journey. Finally, at the top of your body lies your head. This is where you can see the beaming smile. Not only is your smile exuding confidence, but your eyes are showing your true character now as well. You're nourishing yourself and taking care of yourself in the way that you deserve to be loved. You recognize that losing weight isn't something that just makes you look good. Losing weight is an important part of life because we need to be healthy. You deserve to feel good all the time. It's not just a matter of looking good in a bikini.

You're able to walk up a set of stairs without running out of breath. You can have a little bit of ice cream or cake or other indulgent things here and there because you have that powerful self-control. You're able to walk into any store you want and know that you can find something that fits. You're no longer embarrassed or afraid of what other people might think of your body. You can jump into a pool in a swimsuit anytime without thinking twice about what others are going to think. It's not a matter of just fitting into a certain-sized clothing item. You have done this because it makes you feel good from the tip of your toes to the top of your head. You are smiling all the time without even realizing it. This is so powerful.

It's something that you never would have imagined. You thought that you can only achieve something so incredible in a fantasy, but you look in front of you now into the mirror and see that this is exactly what you want. Everything that you have ever desired is in your hands. You are able to give this gift to yourself. Nobody else has ever done something so nice for you. You take care of yourself. You choose a healthy lifestyle because it's going to help you live longer and live happier. You are an incredibly important person in your life. You are your biggest role model. You are able to get the things that you want now because you know that you deserve them. You don't wait around for the right moment. You take your life by the head and run with it.

There is nothing that is going to kill your confidence. Now, you might still have certain goals for your body and want to lose more weight, but overall, you feel incredible.

You've seen your future, and it is bright.

You are beaming with everything that you could ever want. You open the door again and decide to walk towards the chatter. It grows as you approach large wooden carved double doors. Once again, you reach your hand out to the brass handle.

You open the doors, and there it is a huge group of people that love you. They begin applauding, all smiling, with joy spreading across their faces. You manage to bring all these people here, and they're ready to celebrate you.

After hours of hard work in the gym, going for walks and doing other exercises, topped with eating healthy and limiting portions, you are able to create this life. It wasn't always easy, but looking back now, you see just how simple it is to achieve these incredible feats.

You take a step in, and everybody simply gives you a handshake or a pat on the back. They smile and lift their drinks up to you, acknowledging all of the hard work that you put in. Everybody knows that this isn't something simple. You can see on their faces that they might even want it themselves, but they didn't have the strong willpower that you had. You were able to create this incredible life for yourself. You've managed to get everything that you could have ever wanted. No longer is it a fantasy. This is exactly what is needed for your confidence. You are filled with joy. Now that you've seen this visualization, you understand that you can see the future. This weight loss journey is going to happen so quickly. Before you know it, you will be the one walking through this mansion. Notice your breathing once again.

Breathe in for one, two, three, four, and five, and out for five, four, three, two, and one.

You are completely at ease. You walk up a set of stairs and look down and see everybody cheering for you.

You are going to be able to reach new

milestones with ease. Everything is calm around you. There is nothing that is giving you stress or anxiety. You have seen the castle of your future life. You know exactly what you need to do to get back to this place. It feels so natural because you can see it right in front of you. It might seem like a far time from now, but you recognize just how quickly it can happen when you take yourself back to this castle. When you were afraid of what your results might be or anytime you're feeling discouraged, you can come back to this castle. One day you will really be in a place like this, and instead of looking to the future, you'll be able to look to the past. The past will seem so much closer than the future ever does, and this is what is going to make your weight loss journey feel so rapid. Don't look to the future and what is to come. Instead, look at the past and remember all that you have already done. This is how you're going to make your weight loss feel quick so that you're not constantly sad about getting results that you might not have been expecting. You have your dream castle. You have a safe place that you can always revisit. Slowly drift away into sleep now as you remember this.

Feel your body become more and more relaxed. You are sinking deep into your comfortable bed or couch. Nothing around you is causing stress or anxiety. You are completely at ease, happy, and peaceful. You are mindful in this moment, and nothing scares you.

Breathe in for one, two, three, four, and five, and out for five, four, three, two, and one.

We are going to count down once more, and as we do, you're either going to drift off to sleep or move on to another meditation. You know exactly what you have to do to get the quick and easy natural weight loss results that you want for a better life. Don't forget your castle and the reality that awaits you.

Twenty, nineteen, eighteen, seventeen, sixteen, fifteen, fourteen, thirteen, twelve, eleven, ten, nine, eight, seven, six, five, four, three, two, and one.

Chapter 2: Natural Weight Loss Meditation

In this meditation, we are going to be taking you through a mindset that will help the weight loss process feel more natural. Rather than choosing risky diet plans or other things that could harm your body, you will recognize the way that you can work with your natural systems in order to get the things that you want. This weight loss meditation is going to be another visualization exercise that makes it easier for you to relax and accept that your body is going to help you in this process.

Meditation for Natural Weight Loss

You are completely relaxed now. You are in a comfortable place where you feel natural and at ease. We often find ourselves in situations that aren't always natural to us. Maybe you feel uncomfortable at your work office, or perhaps riding the train on the afternoon commute makes you feel out of place. You are not in that mindset now, however. You are in a completely peaceful and serene setting. Nothing around you is distracting whatsoever. You have everything that you could ever need right in this moment. You are making sure that your body is stretched out and that you are at ease. You are perfectly centered in this moment. Your eyes are closed, and your breathing is regulated.

Notice now how the breath comes in and out of your body. This is one of the many natural processes that we go through throughout our entire lives. You need oxygen to come into your body because it spreads to every last part. It goes straight to your brain, to your stomach, and all the way down to your tippy toes. This oxygen moves everything throughout your body naturally in order to ensure that you have consistent blood flow. It is the life source of your entire existence. Regulate your breathing.

Now breathe in through your nose and out through your mouth. This helps create a constant current. It makes you feel more regulated and provides a consistent pattern to your brain. This helps you focus easier so that you aren't hung up on the mega anxieties that normally consume all of your thoughts and emotions. Breathe in for five and out for five. We are going to count down from 20. When we reach one, you will be completely relaxed and calm, there will be no thoughts in your mind, and you will only see black in front of you. You are going to be in a peaceful void, where there are no distractions.

Twenty, nineteen, eighteen, seventeen, sixteen, fifteen, fourteen, thirteen, twelve, eleven, ten, nine, eight, seven, six, five, four, three, two, and one.

You feel fresh and rejuvenated. You are a natural being that doesn't have anything to worry about. You are part of the earth. We have every element within us. We have the earth from the food that we eat. We have the air from the oxygen that we breathe. We have the fire from the sun that beams down from the sky and the way that we generate heat within our bodies. We have water, which makes us up. It is who we are. Every single part of us contributes to one of the main elements. We are able to be a natural part of this earth. We share so many characteristics with other natural living things as well. We are connected to this place that we were born. It is the only place you have ever been and will likely be the only place that you will ever be.

This is an incredibly powerful reminder of who and what we are. We are individual beings, but we are also part of an overall life force. We play a vital role in keeping things going. We are an active member of our community that contributes to other people. Even if we don't have any monetary connections, we still influence people on a daily basis. Just a simple conversation alone can be the beginning of something greater. You are a natural being on this earth, and you deserve everything that comes your way.

You are natural, and you are calm. You let go of the stress that has been holding you down. This stress comes from work, from money, and from our different relationships. You no longer have to let stress be something that controls your life. You feel at peace because you know that this is what you deserve. There are always going to be new tasks that you can finish, but you recognize now that putting yourself first is what's most important.

It is like the analogy of riding an airplane. When the oxygen masks drop down in case of an emergency, you should put your own mask on first. If you spend your time putting masks on other people instead, by the time you make it back to yourself, you will have run out of oxygen. We cannot do this in our daily lives. We need to put ourselves first, and that includes our health. Your health is one of the most important things that you will ever have. You will always have certain things that are out of your control.

For example, we can't always help it if a sick

child that we run into passes their cold on to us. Sometimes we get into a certain accident that we could not have prevented. Our ancestors might pass down genetic conditions to us through our DNA, and that is out of our control as well. What we have control over, however, are other aspects of our lives. We can prevent the risk of heart disease by living a healthy lifestyle. We can regulate our eating habits if we run into an issue with our weight. If we struggle with diabetes, we can also do something about that as well. We have to be more recognizing of the way that we influence our health.

Breathe in. Now as you notice the fresh and rejuvenated feelings that you have surrounding your body, breathe in for one, two, three, four, and five, and out for five, four, three, two, and one.

Everything that you will ever need to lose weight and be healthy already exists inside of you. When you do start to lose weight, your body knows exactly how to process this. Your body is equipped with everything that is needed to help you lose weight. When you limit your food intake, then your body will revert to the fat that you have stored. When you exercise more, then your body knows it should burn more fat in order to provide it with the right amount of energy.

Your body is literally built to help you lose weight. You will know exactly how to do this naturally. You don't need to look at outside sources like surgery or risky diet plans. Breathe in now as you feel how your body naturally works with you. Your body will tell you what it needs and what you might be doing to hurt it. For example, if you are constantly starving yourself because you're trying to lose weight, your body is going to get sick. It's going to let you know that it needs to eat and cause you pain in your stomach. Your body will also listen to what you tell it to do. Breathe in now and realize just how much influence you have over your body.

Breathe in for one, two, three, four, and five, and out for five, four, three, two, and one.

Your thoughts are floating away. Now you understand that it's important to self-reflect and recognize our strengths and weaknesses so that we can mentally grow. But in this moment, you are letting your mind go blank. You don't need to think about anything other than relaxing right now. Relaxing is going to be the way that you can lose weight naturally. You'll be able to avoid the urge to binge-eat. Exercising won't give you as much anxiety if you approach it with a stress-free mindset.

Losing weight naturally is focused on stress. Let's do a visualization exercise now to help you reduce your stress, so you can feel more natural and healthier. We are going to help you connect back to the earth so that you can really recognize the way that you play a role in the world.

You will understand your powerful influence. Breathe in for one, two, three, four, and five, and out for five, four, three, two, and one.

In front of you, you can start to see what looks to be a gravel path. This path is surrounded by different pieces of green life poking through. Some of it has been worn away because you can see that many travelers have crossed over this gravel path. A few trees dot the sides as well, their leaves casting shadows onto the ground.

You take a few steps forward and feel as the gravel crunches beneath your feet. You continue to walk forward and notice all of the wildflowers and other life that is passing around this natural system. You are part of this now. You are influencing the way that some of the bugs or the birds might fly. You walk down the path and disturb a little bird that had been resting on the side. Of course, you didn't do this on purpose. But this bird is not conditioned to be close to humans, so it gently flies away, higher to a tree. If you had not crossed this path, this bird would not have flown up to the tree. You have indirectly changed the course of this bird's life. It might alter the way that it flies later in the day, or perhaps it goes for food that it wouldn't eat had it not flown there originally.

You are incredibly powerful in this way. You have the ability to change things naturally.

You continue to walk forward, noticing that there's a little stream emerging on the side of the path as well. You can hear the water running over the different rocks. You take a step off the trail so that you can look down into the stream now. You see so many little fish swimming against the stream. There are some lily pads with frogs hopping around on top, and some birds fly down quickly to take a swoop out of the water. You gently throw a little rock across the top of the water; it skips effortlessly.

Some of the fish notice the rock and swim away, a little scared. In this way, again, you were reminded of just how much power you have over the system. You can indirectly change things or directly alter the course of some of the other life around you. You continue on the path now and notice that there's a little hill going up. Even though the other side of the path is flat, you decide to take the hill. You don't know what's waiting on top, and though it might be a little bit more of a strenuous walk, you decide to take intrigue over ease. You start to walk up the path and notice that you're breaking a sweat.

You can feel the strain on your legs as you walk up the incline. This does not hurt you. This just reminds you of just how strong your body is. This path is not designed for somebody to be able to easily walk up it right now, but you are doing it. Though you feel a little bit of strain, it just reminds you of just how powerful and strong you are. You feel as little beads of sweat drop down across your forehead, but it does not make you uncomfortable. It is just a reminder of the way that our bodies naturally work to help us.

When our bodies start to sense that we might be putting ourselves through something a little bit or challenging, it will come in and help in any way that it can. It provides you with water naturally to help you hold down as you walk through this process.

You notice the way your heart beats faster as you continue to walk as well. Everything you put your body through has a response that will be in your best interest. Your body is always working for you, never against you.

We have to recognize this. It is a reminder that you should not punish your body; you should only help it. You are a team. Every single part of your body works together in your favor, and the goal at the end is to make sure that you are taken care of. Your body is going to do whatever it has to do to ensure that these needs are met. You continue to walk up the hill, and you notice that there's a large grassy patch in front of you. You walk to this grassy patch and see that there is a break in the trees, giving you a gorgeous view of the mountains. You see that there is a blanket laid out on the grass along with a picnic basket. You sit down on the grass and open the basket, seeing an array of incredible fruit inside. You still feel a little bit of the sweat on your body, but you are completely relaxed now. There is no strain that you're putting your body through any longer. You have walked up this hill, and now you have the reward of the beautiful view in front of you. You have done everything in order to feel healthy in the end. You have worked with your body to give it incredible results.

Take a moment before you dig into this picnic basket to start to breathe again. Notice the way that the air travels in and out of your body. Breathe in for five and out for five, in for five and out for five.

Breathe in for one, two, three, four, and five, and out for five, four, three, two, and one.

You look ahead and see larger mountains. You already made it up one hill, and you're rewarding yourself now with this little relaxation period. It wasn't easy to go up the hill, but you recognize that it was incredibly worth it. You could have continued on to the flat path and the one that was a little easier, but it would not have given you the incredible things that you see in front of you now. You could have chosen to just simply go the way that everybody else does, but now you have a unique experience that not everyone can say that they have given themselves the chance to be a part of.

You recognize the way that you can naturally lose weight in this process. You can work with your body to get the results that you want. You are part of nature, and by recognizing this, you're making it easier on yourself to actually lose that weight. In the end, this is so rewarding.

Now you are at the top of the hill, and you can look down and see the journey that you have gone through. It is a metaphor for your weight loss journey. Yes, it will be very hard, and there will be times when you have to push through and climb the hills that you don't want to. However, once you do make it to the top of the hill, you can look down and see how far you've come. You'll be able to look down and see that it wasn't even that hard in the end; you'll be able to recognize that it is only going to be downhill from now to get back to where you started. It will be an easy downward incline, and that will always be simpler.

The beginning of your weight loss journey is like walking uphill. This is the part where you're going to have to keep pushing through, even when you might feel discomfort. Walking downhill is like keeping up with the weight. After you've made your weight loss goals, you'll be able to keep up with fat by exercising and eating healthy, and it will be so much easier later on than it is in the beginning. You recognize this now. You will be able to come back to the spot as well, and it will be even easier because you're prepared for the incline.

You look out through the break in the trees again and see the mountains in the distance once again, really appreciating their size. There are even bigger mountains, and you recognize that these represent even bigger goals. You plan on climbing these mountains one day — not today, of course, because you are resting and enjoying. However, you have set these bigger goals for yourself because they will have bigger rewards. The mountain will be harder to climb, but the view at the top is going to be more worth it than the smaller mountains. This is an exact representation of the weight loss journey that you're going to go through.

You reach into the basket and pull out a fresh apple. You take a bite and feel as the juices start to flow into your mouth. You crunch down, breaking through the skin and the bits of the apple. Isn't it incredible that something so sweet and delicious is grown so naturally?

You are now able to recognize the delicious flavors that await within natural food. We have been conditioned to eat so many things that are overly indulgent. We have incredibly sweet candies and incredibly greasy foods that give us instant gratification. They are not natural, however, and when we constantly overload our senses like this, we can't appreciate the smaller flavors. You understand now that it's easier to separate yourself from these more intense foods and choose something natural. This provides your body with hydration. It makes you feel cleansed and pure.

You set the apple down, knowing that you don't even have to finish it. You can throw it into the grass, and it will simply become a part of nature. Other animals can come up and chew on it or even make it their home. This is the way that you can contribute to nature. You don't have to finish your food, and you don't have to feel guilty about it when you are constantly eating something so natural. You lay back on the blanket now and look up at the sky. There are a few clouds passing but nothing too intense. These clouds represent what might be blocking the sun.

The sun is your passion, your energy, and your desire to lose weight. Your negative thoughts are simply going to be the clouds. It's okay, and it's perfectly fine to have a few clouds here and there. Of course, that's inevitable. However, a constant thick layer of clouds isn't going to let the sun shine through. It is going to be a constant gloomy storm. Don't let your clouds create a storm. Let these clouds simply pass by in the sky. Every once in a while, they might block the sun, but after a few seconds, they move so the sun can shine bright again. Let this be how you think. It will be the way that passion is created within you and motivation thrives. You close your eyes now and start to drift away. You are completely relaxed and at ease. You are enjoying this moment and soaking up the sun at the end of your journey. Focus on your breathing once again. Breathe in for five and out for five. As we count down from twenty, you will either drift off to sleep or move on to the next meditation. Twenty, nineteen, eighteen, seventeen, sixteen, fifteen, fourteen, thirteen, twelve, eleven, ten, nine, eight, seven, six, five, four, three, two, and one.

Chapter 3: Weight Loss Hypnosis

This hypnosis is going to be a way that will validate your weight loss goals. You will be able to recognize how relaxing and being peaceful throughout the weight loss process makes it easier to keep the pounds off. Keep an open mind with this, and remember to let thoughts flow naturally into your brain as if they were your own.

Hypnosis for Natural Weight Loss

You know how to relax your body. You are an expert at making sure that your limbs can hang freely without tension. We need to let our minds relax now.

Don't just let your body feel like jelly floating through water. Let your mind be as malleable in this process too. With hypnosis, you have to let others into your head for just a moment. So allow your thoughts to flow freely and don't put any pressure on yourself to think a certain thing. Focus now on your breath.

Breathe in for five and out for five. Breathe in through your nose and out through your mouth. This is a way that's going to help make sure that you are focused on healthy living. Breathe in for one, two, three, four, and five, and out for five, four, three, two, and one.

Now we're going to do something a little different. Breathe in for five and then out for one long second. This time, we're only going to breathe in and out through your nose. Breathe in through your nose for one, two, three, four, and five, and out for one and a long and forceful breath.

You are slowly breathing in new air, and then you forcefully push it out as fast as you can. Breathe in for one, two, three, four, and five, and out for one with a quick snap. This way, you focus your breathing and make it easier for the air to flow in and out of your body.

You are going to want to snap your attention on nothing. You can look ahead of you now, but make sure that you get all of your sights out. On the count of three, you're going to snap your eyes closed and also breathe out at the same time.

So look around you and breathe in for one, two, three, four, and five. Now quickly shut your eyes and breathe out in one long breath.

You can go back to regular breathing now but continue to focus on breathing in through your nose and out through your mouth. Try to do it in a pattern of five, but don't get too hung up on the strict structure. Instead, you'll want to focus on letting your thoughts come into your brain as if they were your own.

Keep your mind focused and breathe in. In front of you, in your mind, only with your eyes closed, see the emergence of a spinning wheel. This wheel has nothing special about it. It is simply silver with rubber tires, and it is spinning fast. It is not attached to anything. It is simply a spinning wheel. It spins faster and faster and faster. Stare directly at the silver center. Notice how it continues to cycle through quickly.

Now that tire is turning into a circle of water. The water is flowing around as if it were a washing machine with water being spun in a circle.

The water is spinning and spinning. It is splashing against itself, but it is all still contained within this one simple silver circle. Continue to look at the center. There is nothing else around; everything is black. Notice this silver spinning water. It goes over and over and over in a simple cycle in a simple loop. Focus on the center again as we count for your breathing. Breathe in for one, two, three, four, and five, and out for five, four, three, two, and one.

Suddenly, on the count of three, this spinning cycle is going to snap into every corner of your mind. You are going to be engulfed in this spinning water.

One, two, and three.

You are now in the water. You see around you that you are on a calm beach. The water is not spinning anymore and is completely serene and clear. You walk towards the edge of the beach. You see it now that the water is slapping against the shore. This is the way that it was spinning around in circles in your mind.

No longer is it spinning now, and it is simply a normal ocean slapping against the beach. You can feel the water dripping off your skin, but the sun above you is already drying out. The sun is a vibrant yellow, and it casts a warm glow over your body. The sun kisses you at the top of your head and spreads down all the way to the tip of your toes. You look down at your feet and see that they're submerged in the sand. There is still water gently coming over and washing against your feet. You move your toes upwards, and they break through some of the sand, only for it to quickly form over them again. As the water smooths it out, you look ahead of you and breathe in again. You breathe in for one, two, three, four, and five, and out for five, four, three, two, and one, and notice all of these smells that come in with that. You breathe again for one, two, three, four, and five, and out for five, four, three, two, and one. You feel refreshed, energized, and free.

You are natural, pure, clean, and clear. You are part of this beach now with your feet stuck in the sand. You are like a tree with roots deep under the surface.

You decide now to sit down. You let your bum sink into the sand a little bit more as well. Water continues to emerge around you now like a warm blanket, all the way up to your hips. It keeps you feeling completely centered and pure on the now.

You look around you, to your right and left, and see that there are plenty of rocks. These, of course, don't hurt you. They just simply are part of the sand. You dig your fingers into the sand, a little bit feeling the cold packed down underneath the initial warm on the top of the surface. You dig out a rock and see that it is flat and smooth. You clear a little bit of this rock off using water as it passes over. You throw the rock quickly and sharply against the top of the water and watch as it jumps. It was a nice skipping rock that effortlessly glided across the top.

You do this a few more times with other smooth and flat rocks that surround you. It is a reminder of how you can manipulate nature.

The water is getting higher and higher now, and you are chest-deep in the water. It is perfectly warm and calm, bringing plenty of waves back to the surface. You want to feel the sun on your skin again now, so you decide to stand up.

You walk across the sand, now in the dry area. Sand begins to stick to your legs, but still, it is nice and warm. You walk across, feeling your feet sink deep in. Each new step you take, the bottom of your foot is hot from the surface of the sand. It adjusts quickly as it sinks down, and you feel a sensation over and over again as you continue to walk. You see ahead of you that there is what looks to be a sandcastle. As you get closer and closer, you see that there is no castle at all. It is simply a wall that somebody has built with the sand. You decide to walk all the way through this wall now.

No longer is there something that is going to block off part of the beach. It was simply made by sand, so it was easy for you to destroy with your feet and legs only. As you walk through this section, you recognize that this is a representation of the walls that you have built around yourself. No longer are you going to let yourself be afraid of the things that you want. You can't just be comfortable with the situation you're in anymore. Being comfortable does not always mean being happy. You want to be able to feel completely fresh and pure. You're not attached to the things that you used to be or the person that used to keep your mind stuck in the same situations over and over again.

You sit in the middle of the now-destroyed wall and look out on the beach again. The sun continues to send warm feelings all across your skin.

You breathe in deeply, feeling this ocean air fill your body once again. These oceans are responsible for so much. They are the life force that keeps everybody moving. We take fish from the ocean, and it helps us travel and carry things across waters. You breathe. All of this is a reminder of the incredible world that you're a part of.

While your problems and issues are valid, this is also a reminder of how small some things that seem like such big deals to us really are in the grand scheme of things. There is a great and powerful force that exists just within the world alone.

You are an important part of this, and it is a reminder of the incredible and powerful person that you are.

The sun is setting, so you decide to go for one last and final dip before you don't have the chance anymore. You don't want to swim in the dark, so you decide to wade in a little bit and get your last dose of ocean water right now. You walk in, and the water is all the way up to your hip. You can look down and see the ocean floor because the water is so clear.

You don't really see any fish, but you can see the old shells left over by different crabs or other ocean critters.

You walk a little bit further, and now the water is up to your chest. The waves are so gentle you barely feel them. It's almost as if you were in a deep and warm bath because the water is so relaxing.

You decide to lift your legs up now. Floating on top of the water, you simply move around, letting the waves take you where you need to go. If you go out too far from the shore or off to the side too much, you can gently guide yourself back to where you want to be with a simple arm or leg movement.

You are simply free in the water, almost as if you're flying through the sky. There is no gravity in this moment. You breathe in and out, in and out. The water is surrounding you now. A few droplets will get on your face here and there as the water continues to splash around you, but nothing too extreme.

You close your eyes for just a moment, letting water wash over your face. You are clean, pure, natural, and energized in this moment. Breathe in for five and out for five. Breathe in for five and out for five. Everything around you is turning black. Darkness begins to consume you once again, and you realize you are now back in your bed on the couch, ready to start a new life.

You are pure, energized, and prepared. As we count on from 20, you will be out of this hypnosis. You can then either drift asleep or move on to another mental exercise.

Twenty, nineteen, eighteen, seventeen, sixteen, fifteen, fourteen, thirteen, twelve, eleven, ten, nine, eight, seven, six, five, four, three, two, and one.

Chapter 4: Weight Loss Affirmations

Affirmations are verbal statements that help us to affirm something we believe. So often we say negative affirmations to ourselves without even realizing it. Recognize those negative thoughts and replace them with the positive affirmation that we have listed below. Repeat these to yourself on a daily basis. Write them down on a piece of paper or have notes with them on them that you leave throughout your house. Remember to practice your breathing exercises that we have learned through the other mindset exercises and keep an open mind as always.

Affirmations to Lose Weight Naturally

Losing weight is more than just looking good to me. I understand that I need to live a healthy lifestyle to feel better all of the time..

I know how to lose weight, and actually, I choose to do this in a natural way because it helps me be healthier. I know exactly what I need to do in order to get the things I deserve from this life.

I am capable of reaching all of the goals that I set for myself, and I am the one who decides what I do next with my life.

I recognize that it's important for me to be patient throughout this process. I am able to wait for the results because I know that I will get everything that I want in the end. I do not punish myself because I don't achieve a goal as fast as I had originally hoped. I nourish myself throughout this process. I constantly look for ways to encourage myself and build my self-esteem because I know that is what is going to help me feel the best in the end. I am able to control my impulses. I know how not to act on my greatest urges. I recognize the methods that will help me to enable myself to work harder in the end. I am happy because I know how to say no.

I am able to turn away when I'm confronted with an impulse. I am stronger than the biggest cravings that I have. I am proud of my ability to have a high level of willpower. I trust myself around certain foods and recognize that what tempts me does not control me.

I look to the things that I already have in my life instead of only paying attention to things that I don't have.

This is the way that will help me better achieve everything that I desire. I do not allow distractions to keep me from getting the things that I want. I am able to stay focused on my goals so that I can create the life that I deserve. In the end, even when I am tempted by something or somebody else, I know how to push through this urge and instead focus on my goals. I will wait for everything. Love is coming to me because I know that, when it does, I will feel entirely fulfilled. I am enjoying the journey and the process that it takes to get the body that I want. I recognize that small milestones are worth celebrating.

I do not wait for one big goal to be reached in order to be happy with myself. I look for all the methods needed in order to achieve greatness in this life. I understand that a temporary desire to eat something unhealthy is not worth giving up all of my goals. I know how to distract myself from my biggest cravings so that I can do something healthy instead. I recognize that doing something small is better than doing nothing at all. Even on the days that I don't want to go to the gym, I do something at home to work out so that I can at least accomplish something minor.

Just getting started is the hardest part for me, but I know how to work through those feelings now. I am emotionally aware of what might be holding me back so that I don't allow myself to be tempted by distractions.

I control my feelings and my urges so that I don't do anything that I regret. I am happy because I am knowledgeable about the things that make me who I am.

I am forgiving of myself when I do act on an impulse. I don't punish myself or deprive my body of the basic things that it needs just because I did something wrong. I sacrifice certain things that I want but never to a point where I cause punishment or torture on myself. I am successful because I am dedicated. I have strong willpower because I am successful. I move through my life with gratitude and always look to appreciate the things that I have around me. I can pick myself up when I'm feeling weak.

I am appreciative of even the hard parts of my life because they create the person that I am. I am an important and powerful person. I have control over my body, and nobody else does. I recognize my weaknesses, but in the same breath, I am very aware of my strengths. I balance my life with these things. I empower my strengths and thrive when I am in an environment that helps me grow. I recognize my weaknesses, and I always look for ways to turn them around in order to live more happily and healthily after. I cook meals for myself because it makes me feel healthier and stronger in the end.

I am going to get the dream body that I want because I am able to recognize things that might be healthy or unhealthy for me. I move my body at least once a day. I always feel better after I agree to a workout rather than if I try to avoid one. I am able to give myself rest when I need it. I don't push myself when I'm too stressed out because I know that this isn't going to help me get the things that I want.

I am able to always find motivation and passion within myself. I set my own goals, and I set newer and bigger ones after I achieved ones that I already completed. I do not procrastinate with my goals. I know exactly what I have to do every single day to reach these goals, and I always look for ways to go above and beyond as well. I am constantly improving the methods that I use to live a healthy lifestyle. I self-reflect productively so that I can find real solutions to any issues that I might face. I don't let what other people think take over how I see myself. I am not afraid of judgment from other people because I know that not everything negative that somebody thinks about me is something that is true.

I make the right decision for my body. I understand that even if I make wrong decisions sometimes, they all play a vital role in making me the person that I am today. These struggles are something that I had to undergo in order to become the powerful individual that I am.

I am constantly losing weight because of all this dedication and passion. I feel lighter, happier, and healthier. I am free. I am pure and clean. I am collected and calm. I am peaceful, and I am happy. I heal myself through my weight loss. I take everything bad that I did to my body in the past and turn it into something good, as I exercise and make healthy choices. I am always getting closer and closer to the things that I want. I'm focused on pushing through my biggest setbacks in order to achieve the things that I deserve. I do not sit around and fantasize about what I want anymore. Instead, I know exactly how to get this. I believe in myself because I know that this is going to be the most important part of my journey. I trust my ability to actually lose the weight, and I'm not afraid of what will happen if I don't. I know how to say these affirmations to myself when I feel better.

Other people like being around me. Others recognize my hard work. Others know that I deserve to have good things in my life. When I listened to my body, I am able to thrive. I recognize the things that my body tells me in order to get the best results possible.

I feel good, and I look even better. I look great, and I look incredible because of this. Not only does losing weight help my body to look better, but it also helps my soul, and that is something that can show through so easily to other people. I choose to do things that are good for my body. I value myself, and I have virtue in all that I do. I add value to other people's lives as well. I motivate myself, and therefore, I know how to motivate other people.

I am not afraid of anything. The worst thing that can happen to me is that I stop believing in myself. I will always be my best friend. I will always know how to encourage myself and include confidence in everything that I do. I love myself, and I am proud of the body that I have. I am perfect the way that I am, and I am beautiful. I am happy, I am healthy, and I am free. I am focused, I am centered, and I am peaceful. I am stress-free and thankful. I have gratitude and love. I am attractive, and I am perfect. There is nothing that I need to punish myself for. I accept everything that I am. I love myself. I am healthy. I am happy. I am free.

Conclusion

As you can see from these mindset exercises, a huge part of the weight loss process is going to be mental. You have to allow your mind to be open and let new thoughts come in so that you can reshape the way that you think. For so long, you might have been trapped in mental cycles that keep you in an unhealthy place, unable to keep the weight off.

No longer do you have to endure this kind of physical struggle. You are an incredibly powerful person. You can get everything that you want from this life with a healthy body that you create.

Check out other meditations as well. You could find something more specific such as positive thinking or better sleep so that you can have the triad of a healthy lifestyle.

Heal your mind, body, and soul in order to

get the things that you desire from your life. You might always look for external sources, but remember that you have the power to get everything you want within your own mind.

www.ingramcontent.com/pod-product-compliance
Lightning Source LLC
Chambersburg PA
CBHW031134020426
42333CB00012B/372